The Over-50 Guide
to Psychiatric
Medications

The Over-50 Guide to Psychiatric Medications

Gary S. Moak, M.D.
Elliott M. Stein, M.D.
Joseph E. V. Rubin, M.D.

**American Psychiatric Association
Council on Aging**

Published by the
American Psychiatric Association
1400 K Street, N.W.
Washington, DC 20005

Copyright © 1989 American Psychiatric Association
ALL RIGHTS RESERVED
Manufactured in the United States of America
89 90 91 92 4 3 2 1

First Edition

The paper used in this publication meets the minimum requirements of the American National Standard for Information Sciences—Permanence of Paper for Printed Library Materials ANSI Z39.48-1984. ∞™

ISBN 0-89042-127-7

Contents

List of Figures

Preface

The Over-50 Guide to Psychiatric Medications, written about and for older adults, provides information about psychiatric medications, one of a number of interventions used by psychiatrists and other physicians to treat persons with mental or emotional problems. This book addresses some common questions about the use of psychiatric medications and clarifies the benefits and limitations of treatment with medication. We hope this guide will help you and your family understand what kinds of treatment with medications might be of help. If you are already receiving treatment with medications, we hope that it will help you understand them better.

This guide specifically focuses on

treatment with medication, describing when and why certain medicines may or may not be used. It is designed as a general information guide and briefly answers many questions. This book is not intended to be comprehensive, and its information may not apply to any particular individual. Furthermore, this guide reflects medical practice as the book was written, and new advances in treatment occur all the time. *For specific answers to questions you have about your treatment, ask a psychiatrist, who is a physician with special knowledge of psychiatric medications.*

While we do not discuss other forms of treatment in depth, these other treatments are just as important as medicines in the treatment of older adults. For further information about treatments such as individual or group psychotherapy, family therapy, behavior therapy, or others, it is best to consult your personal physician for a referral to a psychiatrist.

This book is not a replacement for your doctor's skilled care, and you *should not* use it to make changes in your treatment on your own—this would be dangerous.

We hope you will find this book easy to use. It is not necessary to read it all; many readers will find it best to read only selected chapters. The chapters are arranged by type of symptom or disorder. Thus, if you want to know about the treatment of a specific condition, you can look in the Contents for the chapter(s) that fit best. If you are taking a particular medicine and want to learn more about its use, the index of medications in the back of the book will tell you which pages discuss the medicine you have been given.

Even if you are planning to read only about a specific illness or medicine, we recommend that you read

Chapters 1 and 2 as well. These chapters provide important information that will help in the understanding of later chapters. Each chapter contains lists of many of the medicines that make up the groups of drugs being discussed, each identified by both its brand name and its generic name. (Examples of the most commonly prescribed brand names are listed in parentheses after the generic names.) The words printed in bold letters in each chapter are defined in the Glossary for your convenience.

Finally, if you find something you read in this book to be confusing, or if you are not sure how a specific statement may apply to you, the best person from whom to seek an explanation is a psychiatrist.

CHAPTER 1

Mental Health, Mental Illness, and Aging

Just as each of us grows older, our population itself is aging. More people are living longer than ever. The number of people over the age of 60 and the percentage of the population they represent is increasing. People over the age of 85 are the fastest growing group. For most people, living longer means continued opportunity to enjoy a productive, happy life. As people age, though, they often become more susceptible to illnesses that may impose lifestyle limitations ranging from the trivial to the serious. Older people, as those of other age groups, may suf-

fer from mental and emotional illnesses. Such psychiatric disorders, in
particular, may affect the ability to enjoy one's later years.

Unfortunately, misinformation
and misunderstanding about mental
health, mental illness, and aging often
interfere with the delivery of proper
care. Certain important facts should
be appreciated by older people and
their families:

- Not all mental and emotional disorders of later life represent "senility"
  (see Chapter 7).
- Older people often recover or improve; they deserve psychiatric treatment for their mental and emotional disorders as much as anyone
  else. If they are able to get the right
  kind of treatment, they need not
  suffer unnecessarily.

Similarly, other more generally

applicable facts about psychiatric treatment are not widely recognized:

- Seeking help for emotional disorders *is not* a sign of failure. It does not mean you are "crazy" or "senile."
- **Psychotherapy**, the "talking treatment" *is* just as effective for older patients as younger ones; older people *can* change.
- **Psychoactive medications** (medicines used for psychiatric disorders) *are not* just "mind altering drugs" that either "dope you up" or make you a "zombie." In fact, it is partly because a variety of medical treatments for mental disorders *are* effective in older people that there has been such a growth in geriatric psychiatry.

QUESTION: Why can medicines be used to treat emotional or psychiatric disorders?

ANSWER: Because they work! We understand more today about the relationship of the mind to the brain than we ever have before. Many aspects of behavior, such as thinking, feeling, communicating, moving, remembering, planning, etc., depend on various systems in the brain. These brain systems normally are controlled by chemicals that occur naturally in the brain. Psychoactive medications appear to correct problems in the natural biochemistry of these control centers. Many currently available medicines are extremely effective for some disorders, but only partially helpful for others. Much more research is needed to help psychiatrists to both understand the brain better and develop new, even more effective medicines.

QUESTION: What is psycho-therapy?

ANSWER: Psychotherapy—some-times called the "talking treatment" or "talking cure"—is a form of treatment for emotional disturbances. The trained psychotherapist and the pa-tient meet on a regular basis to ex-plore the patient's feelings and experi-ences in the search of understanding and awareness that can ease the pa-tient's pain. As practiced by a psychia-trist, psychotherapy is considered a medical treatment prescribed for med-ically indicated reasons. Therefore, a thorough evaluation by a psychiatrist should precede the initiation of treat-ment. The psychiatrist, who is a physi-cian specially trained in treating men-tal disorders, will determine if psychotherapy is indicated or if medi-cation should be used. Often, the psy-chiatrist recommends both medicine and psychotherapy. Just as no one treatment is effective for all physical diseases, no single form of treatment relieves all mental or emotional disorders.

CHAPTER 2

General Considerations on the Use of Medications in Treating Illness in Older Adults

The use of medication by older people requires special consideration because of the bodily changes that come with aging. Everyone ages differently, leading to much individual variation in the sensitivity to medicines. As the heart, liver, and kidneys mature, medicines tend to remain in the body longer. Thus, for an equal dose of a medicine, the amount in the bloodstream could be higher for an older person than a younger person. For this reason, continued use of medicine by older people, even for a short time, might lead to its accumulation in the body in undesirably high amounts. This kind of accumulation is important since the body's organs, especially the brain, are more sensitive to the effects of medicine.

In addition to changes in bodily function associated with aging, the medical treatment of mental and emotional problems in older people is also complicated by the occurrence of multiple illnesses. Medical problems, in general, are more common in later life. Many physical illnesses can produce symptoms of mental or emotional disturbance. Thus, a thorough general medical evaluation is important as part of the treatment of any psychiatric problem. Further, the use of medication to treat psychiatric problems requires special caution so that preexisting medical problems are not made worse by **psychoactive medicines**. Most older people take at least one prescription medicine; many take two or more. Taking more medications increases the risk of **adverse medicine interactions** when a new medicine is added. An adverse medicine interaction occurs when the actions of two or more medicines combine to produce a harmful effect. *Whenever you receive a prescription for a new medicine, ask your physician about the possibility of interaction with the medicines you already take.* Bring all your medicines with you, or make a list of your prescriptions including the number of **milligrams** and how often the medicine is to be taken.

QUESTION: What are the different effects medicines can have?

ANSWER: All medicines are capable of having many effects, both helpful and harmful. Examples are listed in Figure 1.

Figure 1. **Types of Medication Effects**

- **Therapeutic effect:** The curative or helpful effect of a medication, such as relieving pain, lowering blood pressure, fighting infection, or relieving depression.

- **Side effects:** Undesirable, inconvenient, or occasionally harmful effects that *all* medicines may have at times. Side effects are common and predictable because they are caused by the action of the medicine on other parts of the body. Side effects are more common in older people since their bodies are generally more sensitive to medicine.

- **Adverse reactions:** Unexpected, sometimes harmful effects of a medicine. These are uncommon and generally not severe. They are unpredictable since they reflect the sensitivity of individual people instead of the typical action of the medicine. Allergic reactions are one type of adverse reaction.

- **Toxicity:** The harmful effect of too much of a medicine. Since medicine can accumulate in older people, the risk of toxicity is greater for them.

- **Adverse medicine interactions:** An adverse reaction (defined above) that occurs when the actions of two or more medicines combine to produce a harmful effect. *You should periodically review with your doctor or doctors the need to continue each medicine prescribed for you.* Each of your physicians, if you have more than one, should know about all of your medications, even non-prescription medicines you may use (for example, aspirin or other pain relievers, cold or allergy preparations, vitamin or mineral supplements, and others).

- **Tolerance:** Some medicines lose their effectiveness after prolonged use. Sleeping pills and certain pain medicines are good examples.

Although it may seem that medicine can cause many problems, all medicines are tested extensively before they are approved by the U.S. Food and Drug Administration to be sure there is little chance of severe adverse reactions. Medical research tries to identify newer, more effective medicines with fewer potentially harmful side effects.

QUESTION: How does the doctor decide which medicine to prescribe?

ANSWER: Many factors go into a doctor's decision to prescribe a medicine. Foremost, your doctor will consider your symptoms, diagnosis, and medical history. Your doctor also will take into account the seriousness of the disorder, the need for treatment, and the expected benefits of the medicines available. This will be balanced against the chances of harmful or unpleasant side effects. For each particular medical problem, there is usually a family of medicines available. The various members of a family of medicines (e.g., antidepressants) usually have similar, but not identical, side effects. Your doctor will select a particular medicine from a family of medicines based on your particular needs, as well as on his or her previous experience using the medicines and the pattern of the medication's side effects. Sometimes side effects can be helpful. Your doctor will try to choose a medicine that will maximize the helpful side effects and minimize the unpleasant ones.

QUESTION: How does the doctor know how much to prescribe?

ANSWER: The amount your doctor prescribes will generally fall within the recommended standard **dose** range that is based on medical research with large numbers of people who already have used the medicine. This dose range has to be high enough to allow the medicine to be effective, but low enough to keep side effects and complications to a minimum. Unfortunately, the recommended dose range does not fit every individual. For some medicines, it is possible to adjust the dose, using blood tests that measure the level or amount of medicine in the bloodstream. For others, some trial and error may be necessary to find the right dose for you. For the reasons discussed at the beginning of this chapter, older people often require only one-third to one-half the recommended dose for younger people. Again, because people age differently, some older patients will need higher doses of certain medicines.

QUESTION: Why are medicines prescribed in so many different forms?

ANSWER: A medicine (or drug) is a chemical compound that has a medically helpful effect on the body. Pharmaceutical companies manufacture medicines not only in all different sizes, shapes, and colors, but also as pills, tablets, capsules, elixirs, syrups, and injections. The size or shape of a tablet or capsule does not tell you about the amount of medicine. What is important is the amount of medicine in a particular preparation. The amount or **dose** of a medicine is measured in **milligrams** (mg), a measure of weight. For example, one ounce of water weighs about 3000 milligrams. You can find out your medicine's dosage by looking on the bottle's label. After the name of the drug, it will say the number of milligrams (e.g., "Brand A 100 mg"). However, do not be fooled by this number. The milligram amount of a medicine is not related to how strong it is when comparing different medicines. Two milligrams of one medicine may be stronger than 200 milligrams of another.

Many people are confused about **brand names** and **generic names**. It may be surprising or frightening to discover that the name of the medicine on the pharmacy bottle is different from what your doctor wrote on the prescription. Your pharmacist may have given you a generic form of a brand name medicine. The generic name is the general chemical name of the medicine. The brand name is the name a pharmaceutical company may choose for its product. Usually the brand name and generic forms are medically the same, and some doctors write prescriptions with generic names. Since the generic form is usually less expensive, your pharmacist may give you the generic to help you save money. On the other hand, in some instances generic medicines are not always as effective, and if your doctor indicates a preference the pharmacist will prescribe what your doctor orders. In this book, whenever a particular medicine is mentioned, we will give the generic name, followed by one or two of the most common brand names in parentheses.

This wide choice of medicines helps your doctor tailor treatment to your particular needs. *If the medicine the pharmacist gives you is not what you expected to receive or looks different from what you are used to taking, ask for an explanation.*

QUESTION: What is the best way to take medicine?

ANSWER: Make sure you understand your doctor's directions and follow them. Following the doctor's directions sometimes may not be easy. Poor vision may make it hard to read the directions on the bottle. Forgetfulness may make it hard to remember to take the medicine. Arthritis may make it difficult to get child safety bottles open. Unfortunately, medicine cannot help unless taken according to your doctor's directions. What can be done?

First, *make sure that you can read the directions*. Some pharmacists have large-type labels. Always wear your glasses when you take your medicine. Second, to help yourself remember, *write the directions for each medicine on a piece of paper that you can post on your refrigerator or other location near where you take your medicine*. Other possibilities include putting all your medicines into daily, weekly, or monthly pill dispensing boxes. Your pharmacist sells these, or you can make one by labelling the pockets of an egg carton. Have your family or friends help. Home health care organizations like the Visiting Nurses can help sometimes. *Third, ask the pharmacist for easy-open bot-*

tles if there are no small children in your home. Your doctor may be able to help by simplifying your medication schedule. *If you have problems being able to take a medicine, call your doctor. Do not make changes in how you take your medicines otherwise.* Some general rules about medicines are listed in Figure 2.

Figure 2. **Some General Rules About Medicines**

1. Pay attention to the doctor's explanation and directions.
2. If you don't understand something, ask your doctor.
3. Take medicine according to your doctor's instructions.
4. If you have more than one doctor, make sure each knows about other medicines you are taking, including nonprescription medications.
5. Make sure each of your doctors knows about special conditions you might have such as glaucoma, heart disease, kidney disease, and diabetes.
6. Don't be afraid to ask your doctor to write things down for you if they seem too hard to remember.

CHAPTER 3

The Use of Medications in Treating Mood Disorders

In this chapter, we discuss the use of medicines and electroconvulsive therapy (ECT) to treat severe disturbances of mood (Figure 3). This chapter focuses on **antidepressants, monoamine oxidase inhibitors**, stimulants, and lithium. These groups are listed in Figure 3 and are discussed in separate sections. Our purpose here is to discuss treatments using medicines or ECT. Other forms of therapy that your physician may recommend are important as well. If you have decided to read only this chapter, we suggest that you also review Chapters 1 and 2.

Figure 3.   **Medicines Used to Treat Mood Disorders**

Antidepressant Medications

- Amitryptyline (Elavil, Endep)
- Amoxapine (Asendin, Demolox)
- Desipramine (Norpramin, Pertofrane)
- Doxepin (Adapin, Sinequan)
- Fluoxetine (Prozac)
- Imipramine (Tofranil)
- Maprotiline (Ludiomil)
- Nortriptyline (Aventyl, Pamelor)
- Protriptyline (Vivactil)
- Thyroid (Euthroid, Synthroid, Thyrolar)
- Trazodone (Desyrel)
- Trimipramine (Surmontil)

Other medicines used occasionally in the treatment of mood disorders are listed and discussed in other chapters (see also the Index of Medications).

Monoamine Oxidase Inhibitors

- Isocarboxazid (Marplan)
- Phenelzine (Nardil)
- Tranylcypromine (Parnate)

Stimulants

- Methamphet-amine (Desoxyn)
- Methylphenidate (Ritalin)

Lithium

- Lithium carbon-ate (Eskalith, Eskalith-CR, Lithane, Lithobid, Lithonate)
- Lithium citrate (Cibalith)

What Is a Mood Disorder?

The word *mood* refers to common emotional states we all experience:

sadness, anger, happiness, etc. **Mood
disorders** are illnesses in which a person's feelings are out of proportion to
his life circumstances. Mood disorders
may last for weeks, months, or years
despite events in life that otherwise
would alter the mood state. They include episodic severe depression,
chronic lifelong depression, and **mania**. Mania is a mood disorder characterized by abnormal elation or eupho-
ria (high mood). Some of these
disorders are believed to be brought
about by disturbances in the biological
function of the brain.

   Normal emotional reactions to
life events (such as sadness at the
death of a loved one) are not mood
disorders. Generally, appropriate emotional reactions do not require treatment unless they become unusually
severe or prolonged. In such cases,
psychotherapy may be an effective
treatment.

Many severe mood disorders are associated with disturbances in thinking, behavior, and ability to cope. Mood disorders of this severity usually require treatment with medication in combination with psychotherapy. In older patients, the most prominent features of mood disorders may be anxiety, agitation, fears, social withdrawal, forgetfulness, or physical complaints.

Treatment of Depression

Treatment of Depression with Antidepressants

Severe depression may appear out of the blue, but often *may* be triggered by life stresses or life-changing events such as retirement, physical illness or incapacitation, or death of a loved one. Such depression typically consists of a bad or "black" mood that you can't shake, unjustified feelings of

Medicines in this section include the following:

- Amitriptyline (Elavil, Endep)
- Amoxapine (Asendin, Demolox)
- Desipramine (Norpramin, Pertofrane)
- Doxepin (Adapin, Sinequan)
- Fluoxetine (Prozac)
- Imipramine (Tofranil)
- Maprotiline (Ludiomil)
- Nortriptyline (Aventyl, Pamelor)
- Protriptyline (Vivactil)
- Thyroid (Euthroid, Synthroid, Thyrolar)
- Trazodone (Desyrel)
- Trimipramine (Surmontil)

guilt, hopelessness or worthlessness, and the loss of pleasure in most activities. It is often worse in the morning, and is associated frequently with loss of appetite, insomnia, fatigue, or poor memory and concentration. These typical symptoms may not appear in some older patients with depressive illnesses, however, making it difficult for family members and physicians without special psychiatric expertise with the elderly to recognize the problem. Since depression has many other causes, it is extremely important to undergo a careful physical evaluation to make sure that the depression is not the product of a physical illness such as stroke, heart disease, thyroid gland disease, poor nutrition, or anemia. Other external causes of depression include the use of alcohol, sedatives, or other prescription drugs. *If you are taking one or more medicines for a physical illness and you become severely depressed, ask your physician whether your medicine may be causing you to feel depressed.*

The treatment of some depressive illnesses includes the use of **antidepressant medicines**. These medicines can be very effective when prescribed in proper dosage. They may be prescribed as a single daily dose or be taken as a divided dose at different times of the day.

QUESTION: How long does it take for antidepressants to work?

ANSWER: Unlike many other medicines that produce nearly immediate results, antidepressants usually take several weeks to produce their full effect. Once the medication starts to work, symptoms of low energy, poor sleep, and poor appetite get better first. The sad mood may be the last symptom to be relieved.

QUESTION: Do antidepressants have side effects?

ANSWER: Antidepressants, like all medicines, have side effects. Not everyone who takes antidepressants, however, will experience side effects.

The side effects of antidepressants are summarized in Figure 4.

Antidepressants vary considerably in the number and severity of side effects they produce in different individuals. Therefore, the doctor will select a particular antidepressant that best balances unpleasant side effects with those that actually may be helpful. Thus, for depression associated with severe insomnia, the doctor may prescribe a very sedating antidepressant to be taken before bed; for depression with severe daytime anxiety or agitation, the doctor may prescribe a more calming antidepressant in divided doses taken during the day (e.g., breakfast, lunch, and supper). The doctor will also try to avoid medication that might complicate an already present physical illness. For example, if you already are having trouble urinating, the doctor will tend to avoid prescribing antidepressants that affect the bladder.

Figure 4.   Side Effects of Antidepressants

Common side effects that, if persistent, should be reported to your doctor:

- Lightheadedness or dizziness
- Rapid heartbeat—should be monitored in people with heart disease
- Drowsiness
- Sweating
- Tremor or shaking
- Excessive appetite or craving for sweets
- Disturbing dreams
- Dry mouth—especially if it causes problems with dentures
- Blurred vision—may interfere with reading
- Constipation

- Difficulty urinating
- Loss of appetite—more common with Fluoxetine (Prozac)

Rare side effects that should be reported to your doctor immediately:

- Eye pain—especially in people with a history of glaucoma
- Irregular heartbeat
- Skin rash
- Inability to urinate
- Abdominal pain
- Fainting
- Seizures or convulsions
- Confusion, hallucinations, agitation, disturbed thinking, or forgetfulness

In general, for most patients, antidepressants are safe if they are selected carefully and prescribed on an individualized basis. However, some precautions should be taken. Because antidepressants can affect the heart and blood circulation in some individuals, the doctor may monitor pulse rate and blood pressure sitting and standing, and may check your electrocardiogram. Patients may also take certain precautions:

- *If you are taking any heart medicine, be sure your doctor knows this before you take an antidepressant.*
- *Avoid stopping the medicine suddenly, unless ordered by your doctor.* Some people may experience withdrawal symptoms, including cramps, vomiting, diarrhea, chills, and sweats. These can last only a few days. They are usually mild, but may cause some discomfort.

● *The use of alcohol, sleeping pills, cold or allergy medicines, and some other nonprescription preparations in combination with antidepressants may cause severe drowsiness, making it dangerous to drive or operate machinery.*

● *If you accidentally take an overdose or think you may have taken one, seek medical help immediately.*

QUESTION: What happens if someone's depression doesn't get better, even though they have been taking an antidepressant long enough?

ANSWER: If the necessary laboratory facilities exist in your area, the doctor might order a blood test to check the level of prescribed antidepressant in your bloodstream. If it is not high enough to be effective, the doctor may raise the dose or switch to a different antidepressant. Some people respond to certain medicines but not to others. Unfortunately, today, the only way to make these kinds of judgments is by trial and error.

In certain situations, psychiatrists may try to enhance the effect of the antidepressant by combining it with another type of medicine. When added to antidepressants, low doses of thyroid hormones may bring about an improvement in depressive symptoms in people with normal thyroid gland function. For certain types of depressive illness, combining **neuroleptic medicines** (Chapter 6) with antidepressants can be effective. The addition of lithium sometimes improves the effect of an antidepressant, even in patients who don't have a mood disorder (such as those with manic-depressive illness).

When it appears that a patient's depression is not responding to an antidepressant, many psychiatrists will suggest switching to a **monoamine oxi-**

dase inhibitor (MAOI) or suggest the use of a totally different kind of treatment, electroconvulsive therapy (ECT). In the next two sections, we discuss the MAOIs and ECT.

Treatment of Depression with Monoamine Oxidase Inhibitors (MAOIs)

Medicines in this section include the following:

- Isocarboxazid (Marplan)
- Phenelzine (Nardil)
- Tranylcypromine (Parnate)

Monoamine oxidase inhibitors are a special group of antidepressants that are very effective for severe depression. Some research suggests that they may be especially helpful for people with lifelong depression or depression associated with atypical symptoms, such as cravings for sweets, overeating, sleeping too much, feeling better in the morning and worse in the evening, anxiety attacks, phobia-type fears, and obsessive concerns. MAOIs are also used to treat **panic disorder** (see Chapter 4 for a discussion of treatment of panic disorders). Some research suggests MAOIs may also be effective in treating depression associated with **Alzheimer's disease** and related disorders (see Chapter 7).

In order to take MAOIs, you must follow a special diet that avoids foods high in a naturally occurring chemical called tyramine. Certain medicines that contain related chemicals also have to be carefully avoided. These foods and drugs are listed in Figure 5.

Most patients find that there are only a few items on the diet that they eat or use regularly and that it is fairly easy to maintain the diet. On the other hand, some older disabled patients may require assistance to follow the dietary restrictions.

When a psychiatrist decides to prescribe an MAOI, he will instruct you first on dietary precautions. If you are already taking an antidepressant, the doctor will first lower the dose, then discontinue it altogether and wait one to two weeks before starting an MAOI. Such precautions are taken because antidepressants can interact with MAOIs, causing a dangerous elevation of blood pressure.

Hypertensive crisis is the medical term for such a dangerous and sudden elevation of blood pressure. This is an emergency and requires prompt medical treatment.

Warning: If you are taking an MAOI prescribed by your psychiatrist and you are also seeing another doctor for other medical disorders, be sure each of your physicians knows you are taking an MAOI and understands the necessary precautions to take before

Figure 5.   MAOI Diet and Medications to Avoid

Foods to avoid

- Cheese—except cream cheese, cottage cheese, and ricotta cheese
- Sour cream and homemade yogurt (commercially prepared yogurt is allowed)
- Liver
- Smoked or pickled fish
- Fermented sausages—salami, pepperoni, bologna, summer sausage
- Brewer's yeast
- Banana skins
- Canned or overripe figs
- Fava beans, broad beans, Italian green beans (string beans or baked beans allowed)
- Fermented or aged foods

Drinks to avoid

- Red wine, chianti, sherry
- Liqueurs
- Beer
- Coffee, tea, soft drinks with caffeine

Clear spirits or white wines are permitted in moderation
Caffeine-containing foods or drinks can be consumed in small
amounts
(Consult your doctor regarding acceptable amounts)

Medicines to avoid (Ask your doctor or pharmacist)

- Nonprescription diet pills
- Nonprescription cold or allergy pills

(continued)

Figure 5.   MAOI Diet and Medications to Avoid *(continued)*

- Nonprescription drugs that contain the following chemicals: phenylpropanolamine, phenylephrine, dextromethorphan or ephedrine (these are used in cold tablets, cough syrups, allergy pills, and similar preparations)
- Pain killers other than aspirin, acetominophen (Tylenol, Panadol), ibuprofin (Advil, Datril)
- Prescription amphetamines
- Prescription alpha methyldopa (Aldomet)
- Prescription methylphenidate (Ritalin)
- Prescription oral (by mouth) antidiabetic drugs
- Prescription narcotic pain killers
- Prescription asthma inhalers
- Prescription aminophyllin, epinephrine

*you take other medicines or receive
general anesthesia. Your dentist also
should be told about your MAOI
medication.*

QUESTION: What are the symptoms of a hypertensive crisis?

ANSWER: A hypertensive crisis usually develops suddenly as the result of
a dietary or medication oversight. The
symptoms may include those listed in
Figure 6.

Figure 6. **Symptoms of Hypertensive
Crisis**

- Severe headache—usually in the back
  of the head
- Neck stiffness
- Sensitivity to light
- Nausea and vomiting
- Sweating
- Palpitations
- Rapid or slow pulse
- Loss of consciousness

QUESTION: What should you do if you think you are having a hypertensive crisis?

ANSWER: If the symptoms are mild, you might want to call your doctor first. However, if you are in doubt, or if the symptoms are severe, the safest thing to do is to go to a hospital emergency room as soon as possible. If your blood pressure is dangerously high, the hospital staff physician can provide the necessary treatment to lower it safely and quickly.

QUESTION: That sounds very frightening—why would psychiatrists prescribe MAOIs?

ANSWER: Psychiatrists prescribe MAOIs because they work well for severe depression and offer certain advantages over other antidepressants. MAOIs sometimes work faster, occasionally within a few days. Remember, other antidepressants can take up to four to six weeks to achieve their full effects. MAOIs also have fewer side effects than many other antidepressants. They have fewer effects on the heart and do not as often cause blurred vision, dry mouth, difficulty urinating, forgetfulness, or confusion.

With proper instructions and precautions, hypertensive crises are extremely rare. When your doctor prescribes MAOIs, make sure that you can follow the restrictions, or that you have all the help you need to do so.

QUESTION: What are the side effects of MAOIs?

ANSWER: Since MAOIs often lower blood pressure, light-headedness is a common side effect. If you have high blood pressure and already take anti-hypertensive medication, it may be necessary to lower this medicine when you start taking an MAOI so your blood pressure doesn't get too low. See

Figure 7. **Side Effects of MAOIs**

Common side effects that, if persistent, should be reported to your doctor:

- Drowsiness
- Insomnia
- Loss of appetite
- Fatigue
- Dry mouth
- Dizziness
- Light-headedness
- Weight gain
- Constipation
- Nervousness
- Shakiness

Rare side effects that should be reported to your doctor immediately:

- Skin rash
- Fainting
- Fever
- Blurred vision
- Sweating
- Irritability with agitation or extreme talkativeness
- Problems with sexual functioning
- Severe headaches

Figure 7 for a list of side effects of MAOIs.

MAOIs sometimes cause difficulty falling asleep. For this reason, dosages are often prescribed for the morning hours.

Treatment of Depression with Stimulants

Medicines in this section include the following:

- Methamphetamine (Desoxyn)
- Methylphenidate (Ritalin)

Stimulant medications (also known as psychostimulants) are used commonly to treat attention deficit disorder in children. Occasionally, they are used to treat depression in older people. Stimulants seem to be most helpful in relieving the apathy, withdrawal, and underactivity experienced by some people with severe depression. Since relatively small doses may be effective, these medicines are usually medically safe for older patients.

Treatment of Depression with Electroconvulsive Therapy

In this section, we do not discuss medicines; rather we talk about a safe and effective treatment for depression that may be recommended by some physicians as an alternative or adjunct to medicine. **Electroconvulsive therapy** (ECT) is a physical treatment that works like medicine for severe mood disorders and which may be preferable to medicine for some patients.

ECT is a therapy that works by medically inducing an electrically stimulated seizure. It was discovered by accident many years ago, when physicians observed that some patients with severe mental illness who also happened to have epilepsy temporarily improved after an epileptic seizure. Some older patients who received treatment several decades ago may remember when medicines—insulin or metrazole—were used to induce the seizures. Back then, "shock" treatment was used to treat a number of severe psychiatric disorders.

Today, ECT is used almost exclusively for the treatment of severe depression in patients meeting certain criteria, such as those who 1) have not responded to other treatment, 2) have a prior history of good response to ECT, or 3) cannot tolerate the side effects of antidepressant medicines. For the treatment of severe depression, ECT is extremely effective. As many as 90 percent of severely depressed patients will respond to it. Moreover, it usually works faster than antidepressant medicine and may be safer medically for some older patients.

QUESTION: If this is such a good treatment for severe depression, why does it seem so controversial?

ANSWER: ECT's bad public image is based largely on misunderstanding. Two commonly held myths are that ECT causes brain damage and that it is barbaric. Some elderly patients may have had a bad experience receiving this treatment several decades ago when outdated methods were used. Modern techniques, however, are much more sophisticated and maximize patient comfort.

QUESTION: What does the treatment actually involve?

ANSWER: ECT treatment itself is very brief; it takes about five minutes. Before the treatment, the patient may be connected to a heart monitor, a brain wave monitor, and an intravenous line. Oxygen is given, and then sleep is induced with an anesthetic similar to sodium pentathol, but shorter-acting. A muscle relaxant is given so the seizure does not cause a severe physical convulsion. People with arthritis of the spine may need to wear a neck collar. A short pulse of electricity, lasting about one second, is passed through the head. For a few minutes afterwards, the electrocardiogram is monitored; medications may be given if necessary for disturbances of the rhythm of the heart that occasionally may occur. The treatments are usually given in the morning, on an empty stomach. Within approximately 30 minutes after the treatment, patients are up and around, able to eat breakfast. The treatments usually are given in the hospital every other day. Severe depression typically responds in four to 12 treatments.

QUESTION: Is ECT medically safe?

ANSWER: Yes, ECT is very safe if performed by a psychiatrist who is skilled in its use. A careful physical evaluation is necessary first. This may include a physical examination, routine blood tests, x-rays of the chest and spine, an electrocardiogram, and an electroencephalogram. Additional caution is exercised in the presence of certain medical conditions such as a recent heart attack or certain neurological conditions. Some rare complications can occur. These include bone fractures or a heart attack. Death occurs rarely, in one out of every 10,000 cases.

QUESTION: Can ECT cause brain damage?

ANSWER: There is no evidence that ECT causes brain damage. However, there are some neurologic side effects that people sometimes find frightening. Immediately after the treatment, most people feel groggy for 10 minutes to an hour. There may be a period of confusion for a few hours thereafter. Some people develop difficulty remembering events that occurred during the period in which treatment was received. This usually stops once the treatments are stopped. On rare occasions, it may last for weeks or months. *(Note: While some former patients feel they have had permanent memory problems as the result of ECT, no scientific evidence is available to verify this claim.)*

Treatment of Mania

Information in this section relates to the use of lithium. Other drugs that may be used in the treatment of **mania** also will be mentioned in this section. More detailed discussions of these other medications may be found in other chapters (see the Index of Medications).

Medicines in this section include the following:

- Lithium carbonate (Eskalith, Eskalith-CR, Lithane, Lithobid, Lithonate)
- Lithium citrate (Cibalith)

Mania is a type of *pathological* or *abnormal* mood state. In contrast to depression, it is characterized by a persistently elated or euphoric mood, an abnormal and unrealistic sense of well-being. In many cases, manic patients also experience a mood that is abnormally irritable or angry. The abnormal mood is often associated with other symptoms such as increased energy, decreased need for sleep, hyperactivity, disturbed thoughts, rapid thinking and rapid speech, and impulsiveness. Episodes of mania can last for days, weeks, or months.

Mania may be seen in manic-depressive illness, which psychiatrists now call **bipolar disorder.** In this condition, which usually begins earlier in life, but, on occasion, may start during the senior years, episodes of mania and depression occur in the same person at different times. Older patients are particularly susceptible to an experience of manic behavior as the result of other physical illnesses that affect the brain. These causes include strokes, brain tumors, metabolic disturbances (e.g., hyperthyroidism), seizure disorders, medications (including antidepressants), and ECT. Again, it is extremely important to undergo a thorough physical evaluation to look for these other causes of manic symptoms that, if persistent, would require other treatments.

The principal medication for patients with bipolar disorder is treatment with lithium. Lithium is a chemical element, similar to sodium or potassium. For medical purposes, lithium is given in the form of lithium carbonate (Eskalith, Eskalith-CR, Lithane, Lithobid, Lithonate) or lithium citrate (Cibalith). It is classified as a mood stabilizer, and is effective both for treatment of manic symptoms during acute episodes and as a treatment during normal periods to prevent the return of either manic or depressed moods. Lithium alone, however, is not as good an antidepressant for most people as other medications we have mentioned.

Once a manic episode is diagnosed, treatment with lithium is usually begun. Unfortunately, it generally takes some time for lithium to exert its effect on manic symptoms. Frequently when manic symptoms include severely disturbed behavior that must be controlled quickly, **neuroleptic medicines** are prescribed. These medicines are used for the treatment of severe agitation and disturbed thinking and behavior (see Chapter 6).

Since they often *do* work right away, they can be very helpful during the period before lithium takes effect.

Once the manic or depressive symptoms are under control, lithium may be continued as a *maintenance treatment* to prevent future relapse. During this maintenance treatment phase, neuroleptic medicines, if started earlier, may no longer be necessary. Some patients may need *additional* antidepressant medicine to prevent an occurrence of depression. Once someone's condition is stabilized on lithium, many psychiatrists recommend continuing to take it indefinitely for preventive purposes.

The prescribed dose of lithium is adjusted based on the level of the medicine in the bloodstream, measured by a simple blood test. A typical starting dose for older patients is 150 mg to 300 mg twice a day. Until the symptoms are controlled and the dose is properly adjusted, blood levels are checked frequently. In general, the lithium level should be between .6 and 1.2, but for older patients, levels between .3 and .9 may be sufficient.

QUESTION: What are the side effects of lithium?

ANSWER: The side effects of lithium are listed in Figure 8.

The more common side effects frequently occur when lithium treatment first begins. They usually subside immediately if the dose is lowered. If the dose cannot be reduced, a few other things can be done. A medicine, propranolol (Inderal), is sometimes used to treat the tremor caused by lithium. Sometimes the nausea is less severe if lithium citrate (Cibalith) is used instead of lithium carbonate (Eskalith, Eskalith-CR, Lithane, Lithobid, Lithonate), or if the medicine is taken with tomato juice.

Figure 8.   **Side Effects of Lithium**

Common side effects that, if persistent, should be reported to your doctor:

- Increased thirst
- Increased urination
- Diarrhea
- Mild Nausea
- Fine hand tremor or shakiness
- Dry mouth

Rare side effects that should be reported to your doctor immediately:

- Severe nausea
- Vomiting
- Severe diarrhea
- Irregular or rapid heartbeat
- Muscular weakness
- Drowsiness
- Lack of coordination
- Confusion
- Blurred vision
- Swelling of hands and feet
- Slurred speech

Later side effects, especially the less common ones, may indicate that the lithium level has become too high. They should be reported to your doctor right away. Certain precautions may be taken to avoid high lithium levels. Avoid dehydration. Since lithium may cause increased urination and excessive thirst, some patients need to drink more water while taking lithium. During hot weather or other periods of heavy sweating, extra care is needed to replace fluids. Older patients are more prone to dehydration and sometimes need help to make sure they drink all the extra fluids they need. In extreme cases of excess urination, the doctor may prescribe a thiazide diuretic—a certain type of "water pill"—to lessen the urine production.

Under certain circumstances known to affect the level of lithium in the body, the doctor may order blood tests more often and carefully readjust the dose of medicine as needed. These circumstances include gastrointestinal illness, a change in dietary salt intake, treatment with diuretic medicines ("water pills"), and dehydration.

QUESTION: Doesn't lithium cause serious medical problems?

ANSWER: As with all medicines, lithium potentially can cause adverse effects or medical complications. In addition to the previously listed side effects, lithium infrequently can affect the function of the heart, the kidneys, and the thyroid gland. Thus, as a precaution, the doctor will order an electrocardiogram and blood tests of the kidney and thyroid gland function both before starting lithium and periodically during treatment. If there are medical complications, it may be necessary to stop the lithium.

In some people, lithium will promote decreased thyroid activity. Symptoms which may suggest the presence of this problem are listed in Figure 9.

When lithium is stopped, the thyroid gland returns to normal function. If you develop this problem and lith-

Figure 9.   **Symptoms That May Be Related to Underactive Thyroid Gland**

- Tiredness
- Muscle aches
- Constipation
- Coldness
- Unexpected weight gain
- Dry, puffy skin
- Hoarseness
- Feeling slowed down

ium is clearly helping you, your doctor may decide to continue the treatment and, at the same time, prescribe thyroid hormones for you. Also bear in mind, however, that there may be other causes for the symptoms listed above. Your doctor can conduct an evaluation to identify the particular cause in your case.

QUESTION: What can be done for people who need lithium but cannot take it?

ANSWER: About 30 percent of patients with manic-depressive disorder do not respond to lithium. Of those who do get better, some cannot tolerate the side effects of lithium. Some of these patients can be treated with **neuroleptic medicines** (see Chapter 6). A few other medicines that have been found to be effective for some patients with manic-depressive illness might also be tried. These include carbamazepine (Tegretol), clonazepam (Klonapin), diltiazem (Cardiazem), nifedepine (Procardia), valproic acid (Depakene, Depakote), and verapamil (Isoptin). While these may help some patients, no medicine has ever been proven scientifically to be as effective as lithium.

CHAPTER 4

The Use of Medications in Treating Anxiety Disorders

In this chapter, we discuss the use of medicine in the treatment of anxiety. Although other forms of therapy are important in the treatment of anxiety, our purpose here is to discuss the use of medicine. If you have decided to read only this chapter, we recommend that you review Chapters 1 and 2.

The **antianxiety medicines,** sometimes referred to as **"minor tranquilizers,"** are prescribed commonly for the treatment of symptoms of anxiety (Figure 10). They are recognized to be safe and effective for the short-term relief of severe anxiety associated with

Figure 10.   **Medicines Used to Treat Anxiety Disorders**

- Alcohol
- Alprazolam (Xanax)
- Buspirone (Buspar)
- Clorazepate (Tranxene)
- Chlordiazepoxide (Librium)
- Diphenhydramine (Benadryl)
- Diazepam (Valium)
- Ethchlorvynol (Placidyl)
- Glutethimide (Doriden)
- Hydroxyzine (Atarax, Vistaril)

- Lorazepam (Ativan)
- Mephobarbital (Mebaral)
- Meprobamate (Equanil, Miltown)
- Oxazepam (Serax)
- Pentobarbital (Nembutal)
- Phenobarbital (Luminal)
- Prazepam (Centrax)
- Promethazine (Phenergan)
- Secobarbital (Seconal)

major life crises and are helpful in the psychiatric treatment of a group of illnesses known as anxiety disorders. Antianxiety medicines have been found to be important in the treatment of alcohol detoxification symptoms, as well.

Anxiety is a common complaint of many people, including the elderly. There are many different causes of anxiety, requiring different treatments. Unfortunately, it is also fairly common for older people to receive prescriptions for antianxiety medicines. This practice is troubling since these medicines can be too strong and habit-forming. Moreover, their indiscriminate use can lead to other symptoms such as depression, confusion, memory problems, and disturbed sleep. Therefore, these medicines should be prescribed only by physicians who know when, and for how long, to use them.

What do we mean by anxiety? Anxiety is an inner emotional feeling of tension, nervousness, apprehension, uneasiness, dread, or worry. Associated physical symptoms may include sweaty palms, rapid heartbeat, tightness in the chest, shallow breathing, butterflies in the stomach, diarrhea, and restlessness or fidgeting. Other symptoms that may be misinterpreted as anxiety include tremor (shaking), restlessness, boredom, forgetfulness, depression, impatience, and irritability.

Everyone experiences brief periods of anxiety from time to time in response to life's stresses. Antianxiety medicines *should not* be used for this transient type of anxiety. Treatment may be helpful when anxiety is very severe, long-lasting, or interferes with functioning. Older people may have realistic and legitimately disturbing concerns about such things as loneliness, health, death, retirement, finances, and independence. For anxiety arising from such seriously life-stressing difficulties, psychotherapy, either alone or in combination with medication, or counseling may be effective.

Frequently, anxiety is a symptom of another medical problem. Antianxiety medicines are ineffective in the treatment of medical problems that require more specific treatments. Thus, it is important to see your doctor early for a thorough evaluation. Patients with delusional fears (Chapter 6) or depression (Chapter 3) may appear to be extremely anxious. For such patients, treatment with antianxiety medicines will be less effective; they should receive neuroleptics or antidepressants instead. Many other conditions, such as low blood sugar, overactive thyroid, other glandular diseases, certain heart conditions, and menopause, may produce anxiety as their first symptom. Medicines for other physical and mental illnesses may cause anxiety as a side effect. Finally, caffeine consumption and alcohol abuse are often associated with symptoms of anxiety.

Classes of Antianxiety Medicines

Minor Tranquilizers

Medicines discussed in this section include the following:

- Alprazolam (Xanax)
- Chlorazepate (Tranxene)
- Chlordiazepoxide (Librium)
- Diazepam (Valium)
- Lorazepam (Ativan)
- Oxazepam (Serax)
- Prazepam (Centrax)

Minor tranquilizers are effective and relatively safe medicines and are among the most frequently prescribed drugs in all of modern medicine.

Their popularity is related to their safety and quick action. Unlike some other medicines used in treating mental illnesses (e.g., antidepressants), minor tranquilizers work right away. Their immediate effect, however, also makes minor tranquilizers popular drugs of abuse.

Unfortunately, even when used exactly as prescribed, these safe and effective medicines are associated with potentially serious problems. Each of these problems is more likely to occur and to be more severe in older people. We discuss these problems below.

Side Effects. Although the minor tranquilizers are safe drugs, the occurrence of these side effects may indicate the need to lower the dose or stop the medicine. Thus, *any* side effects should be reported to your doctor. See Figure 11 for the side effects of minor tranquilizers.

Figure 11.   **Side Effects of Minor Tranquilizers**

- Drowsiness or sedation
- Lack of coordination
- Slurred speech
- Depression
- Confusion
- Forgetfulness
- Disturbed sleep patterns
- Bizarre dreams
- Increased sleep-related breathing disturbances (see Chapter 5)
- Dry mouth
- Bitter taste

Note: *Any* side effects should be reported to your doctor.

Tolerance and *Addiction.*
Unlike most of the medicines used in psychiatry, the minor tranquilizers may be addicting. After prolonged use (possibly as short as a few weeks), the body becomes tolerant to the medicine's effect. You may feel the need to take greater quantities of the medicine

to continue to experience an effect from it. Once tolerance develops, failure to continue taking the medicine may lead to **withdrawal** symptoms.

Withdrawal.   Once your body becomes dependent on the presence of a medicine, stopping it may lead to **withdrawal symptoms** (Figure 12). (A common example is the reaction smokers experience when they try to quit "cold turkey.") *If you have been taking minor tranquilizers, sudden cessation may give rise to serious symptoms that may require medical attention.*

Depressant Effects.   Even in moderate doses, minor tranquilizers depress the functioning of the central nervous system, leading to confusion, poor memory, and slowed thinking, which may resemble Alzheimer's disease or other types of **dementia** (see Chapter 7). *When someone taking mi-*

Figure 12.   **Symptoms of Minor Tranquilizer Withdrawal**

- Anxiety—often
  within hours of
  the first missed
  dose
- Agitation
- Confusion or
  disturbed
  thinking

- Insomnia,
  nightmares
- Shakiness
- Sweats
- Fainting
- Convulsions
- Fever
- Sweating

Warning: *Withdrawal symptoms may
be mistaken for the symptoms of anxiety
for which the antianxiety medicine was
originally prescribed. This mistake may
lead to an incorrect attempt at treatment
by raising the dose, further compounding
the problem.* Withdrawal problems generally can be avoided by gradually reducing the dose of the medicine over
days or weeks before halting it
completely.

nor tranquilizers for anxiety develops other mental or emotional symptoms, the minor tranquilizers may be the cause.

Misuse of Minor Tranquilizers.
Many people, including seniors, turn to minor tranquilizers or alcohol to "help them manage" anxiety caused by stressful life events. When supervised by a physician, minor tranquilizers can be a valuable treatment for short-term use. Inappropriately, some patients continue to take these medicines indefinitely. Considerable medical expertise is required to diagnose the causes of anxiety and to prescribe other medically indicated treatments for anxiety such as psychotherapy or behavioral therapy. Anxious patients, in the belief that people should be able to handle all problems on their own, may be reluctant to seek needed help from a psychiatrist. Some people feel there is a stigma attached to both

anxiety *and* psychiatric treatment. Alcohol is more readily available than prescription medicines, and we now know that many more older people have a problem with drinking than was previously recognized.

QUESTION: What can be done for people who are dependent on tranquilizers or alcohol?

ANSWER: Treatment for medication dependence requires close medical supervision and, at least initially, should be undertaken in the hospital. The first step is **detoxification**. In the case of alcohol abuse, minor tranquilizers are actually the recommended medication to accomplish detoxification. During detoxification, the medicine dosage is reduced gradually over many days in a safe, medically controlled way. (Long-term use of narcotic pain medicine may lead to similar addiction problems. In this case, detoxification might be done with other medicines such as methadone, clonidine [Catapres], or naltrexone [Trexan].)

Treating a drug or alcohol problem involves more than detoxification. Being able to "get off" a drug and "stay off" usually requires psychotherapy or other active treatment by your doctor. Programs such as Alcoholics Anonymous and others can be helpful for many older people with alcohol or drug problems. A thorough psychiatric evaluation is also important to diagnose other coexisting mental or emotional disorders. For example, alcohol or tranquilizer abuse may be a person's own attempt to treat depression (see Chapter 3). In this case, treatment for the drug dependency might be ineffective without simultaneous treatment for depression.

Buspirone

Buspirone (Buspar) is a new anti-anxiety medicine with novel properties. It is not chemically related to any of the other groups of medicines used in the treatment of anxiety. It may offer the advantage of being effective without being habit-forming.

Antihistamines

Medicines in this section include the following:

- Diphenhydramine (Benadryl)
- Hydroxyzine (Atarax, Vistaril)
- Promethazine (Phenergan)

The **antihistamines** are a group of medicines commonly used for relief of allergic symptoms and itching. Many are available for this purpose as over-the-counter medicines. The antihistamines exert a mild antianxiety effect that may be helpful in many clinical situations. Their principal advantage, in comparison with minor tranquilizers, is that they are nonaddicting. Unfortunately, they may be very sedating and many have anticholinergic side effects that may be a problem in older patients.

Barbiturates and Other Medicines for Anxiety

Medicines in this section include the following:

- Glutethimide (Doriden)
- Mephobarbital (Mebaral)
- Meprobamate (Equanil, Miltown)
- Ethchlorvynol (Placidyl)
- Pentobarbital (Nembutal)
- Phenobarbital (Luminal)
- Secobarbital (Seconal)

The barbiturates and other medicines discussed in this section are no longer commonly used. Although effective in relieving symptoms of anxiety, their use causes many problems. In addition to producing all of the potential side effects of the minor tranquilizers, these medicines are more powerfully addicting, very sedating, and, in toxic amounts, may dangerously depress breathing. Although the minor tranquilizers are much more frequently prescribed today, many older people who were prescribed barbiturates 20 or 30 years ago may be strongly addicted to them now. This problem is potentially serious since, as the body ages, the margin of safety for these medicines gets narrower, increasing the risks. "Getting off" barbiturates requires the same approach outlined in the section on **minor tranquilizers.**

Using Medications to Treat Anxiety Occurring with Depression

As mentioned before, anxiety may occur as a symptom of depressive illness. In such cases, the most effective approach is to treat the depressive illness (see Chapter 3). When the depression improves, the anxiety goes away. *Antianxiety medicines are generally not good medicines for depression; they may make it worse.* However, since antidepressants take several weeks to have their full effect, some psychiatrists will prescribe both antidepressants and other medicines, such as minor tranquilizers or neuroleptic medicines, for the short-term alleviation of anxiety symptoms.

Using Medications to Treat Anxiety Associated with Disturbed, Irrational Thinking

Disturbances of thinking may lead to false suspicions or fears of harm that cause much anxiety. Treating this type of anxiety involves recognizing and treating the disturbances of thinking. These are usually treated with **neuroleptic medicines** (see Chapter 6).

Using Medications to Treat Panic Disorder

Panic disorder is a type of anxiety disorder in which people experience sudden terrifying panic for no apparent reason. This unpredictable, but recurring, experience may then lead to more continuous anxiety and reluctance or refusal to go out.

For reasons that are not known scientifically, panic attacks often may be controlled by certain **antidepressant**

medicines. Antianxiety medicines may have a temporary calming effect, but they do not *prevent* panic attacks from returning. In the event that an older patient is unable to take antidepressants, two alternative medicines are currently recognized to have *antipanic* effects. These are the MAOI-type antidepressants (Chapter 3) and alprazolam (Xanax), a newer member of the minor tranquilizers.

To summarize, anxiety is a common symptom that sometimes requires medical treatment. The minor tranquilizers are safe and effective for short-term use. When anxiety is more long-lasting or is severe, a psychiatric evaluation is necessary to determine the need for other treatments. Continued long-term use of minor tranquilizers is not appropriate for many people and, if chosen as a treatment, should be taken only under the close supervision of a psychiatrist.

CHAPTER 5

The Use of Medications in Treating Insomnia and Other Sleep Disorders

In this chapter, we discuss medicine commonly identified as sleeping pills. Although other forms of therapy are important in the treatment of sleep problems, our purpose here is to discuss medicines prescribed for sleep (Figure 13). If you have decided to read only this chapter, we recommend that you also review Chapters 1 and 2. Information in this chapter also applies to the antianxiety medicines discussed in Chapter 4.

Insomnia, or difficulty sleeping, is

Figure 13.   Medicines Used to Treat Sleep Disorders

- Alprazolam (Xanax)
- Chloral Hydrate
- Chlorazepate (Tranxene)
- Chlordiazepoxide (Librium)
- Diazepam (Valium)
- Diphenhydramine (Benadryl)
- Flurazepam (Dalmane)
- Hydroxyzine (Atarax, Vistaril)
- Lorazepam (Ativan)
- Oxazepam (Serax)
- Paraldehyde
- Pentobarbital (Nembutal)
- Prazepam (Centrax)
- Promethazine (Phenergan)
- Secobarbital (Seconal)
- Temazepam (Restoril)
- Triazolam (Halcion)

a common problem among older people. It is a complicated problem that has many possible causes. Many older people receive prescriptions for sleeping pills. Although sleeping pills may be very safe and helpful for some types of insomnia, their chronic, indiscriminate use is medically unwise. Just as it is medically unwise to take pain medicine indefinitely without finding the cause of the pain, it is also bad to take sleeping pills indefinitely without finding the cause of the insomnia. Different causes of insomnia may require different, specialized treatment. Sometimes, sleeping pills are an incorrect treatment.

Before we discuss the various causes of **insomnia** that might require treatment, it is important to distinguish abnormal sleeping problems from normal sleeping difficulty. As people get older, they often sleep less soundly. Some people find that in contrast to when they were younger,

Figure 14.　Causes of Sleeping Difficulty in Older Adults

• *Emotional stress:*　Most people have experienced one or more periods of insomnia during stressful times in their lives. Unless prolonged or severe, it usually goes away without treatment.

• *Psychiatric illnesses:*　Sleep disturbance is a common symptom of many psychiatric illnesses. In depression, insomnia may be profound (see Chapter 4). In mania, there is a decreased need for sleep (see Chapter 3).

• *Poor sleep hygiene:*　People often fall into habits that may lead to insomnia such as taking too many daytime naps, smoking or drinking alcohol or caffeine in the evening, and undertaking stimulating chores or other physical activities just before bed.

• *Physical health problems:* Certain physical illnesses may make it hard to sleep. People with urinary problems, who wake up to go to the bathroom, may find it difficult to go back to sleep. Painful conditions like arthritis may keep people awake. Congestive heart failure may cause shortness of breath while in bed. Treatment of these and other physical problems that affect sleep often leads to improved sleep without the need for sleeping pills.

• *Sleep apnea:* This is a sleep-related breathing problem more common in very overweight people. It causes frequent awakening and may lead to excessive daytime tiredness.

• *Leg jerks:* Leg jerks, known medically as *nocturnal myoclonus*, may occur during sleep and lead to awakening.

(continued)

Figure 14. Causes of Sleeping Difficulty in Older Adults
(continued)

• ***Sundowning:*** This is the tendency for some patients with Alzheimer's disease or related disorders to experience severe agitation in the evening, often interfering with sleep and mistakenly being treated as insomnia.

• ***Depression:*** Sleep difficulties are a frequent symptom of severe depression (Chapter 3).

they spend more time in bed, but less time asleep. For some people this may be an unavoidable part of aging. Yet, there are many other causes of insomnia in older people that may benefit from treatment (Figure 14).

QUESTION: When are sleeping pills helpful?

ANSWER: Sleeping pills may be very helpful for severe insomnia associated with serious stressful life crises. Under these circumstances, they are suggested only for short-term use. Collateral psychotherapy may be needed, and may do more than sleeping pills to manage the effects of severe stress. Sleeping pills also may be of temporary benefit to people with insomnia caused by acute physical illness or a flareup of a chronic disorder, such as arthritis. Finally, sleeping pills are sometimes used for the short-term relief of insomnia associated with psychiatric disorders such as depression (see Chapter 3).

QUESTION: What kinds of problems can be caused by using sleeping pills?

ANSWER: Use of sleeping pills may be associated with a number of problems that may be especially severe in older people. Some sleeping pills are sufficiently long-acting to produce "hangovers" the next day. Some are so short-acting that they wear off too soon, causing abrupt awakening in the middle of the night, known medically as *rebound insomnia.* Sleeping pills tend to depress the functioning of the nervous system. This can lead to symptoms of depression, forgetfulness, or confusion that are sometimes mistakenly thought to represent **dementia** (see Chapter 7). Many sleeping pills may worsen sleep-related breathing problems. In turn, this can produce daytime confusion, also often mistaken for senile dementia. Finally, many sleeping pills produce **tolerance**, the basis for physical addiction. When tolerance develops, the body no longer responds to the sleep-producing effect of the medicine. Two things can then happen: either the original insomnia returns or a higher dose of medicine is needed for sleep. The higher the dose taken, the greater the risk of **toxicity** (see Chapter 2). The dose required to produce toxicity in older people is generally lower than for younger people.

Many different types of medicines can be prescribed for sleep. Medicines that bring on sleep are known as **sedative-hypnotics**. This group of medicines overlaps significantly with the **antianxiety medicines**, so additional information about these may be found in Chapter 4.

Benzodiazepines

Medicines in this section include the following:

- Alprazolam (Xanax)
- Chlorazepate (Tranxene)
- Chlordiazepoxide (Librium)
- Diazepam (Valium)
- Flurazepam (Dalmane)
- Lorazepam (Ativan)
- Oxazepam (Serax)
- Prazepam (Centrax)
- Temazepam (Restoril)
- Triazolam (Halcion)

Although some medicines in this group are identified primarily as sleeping pills, others, identified primarily as antianxiety medicines (Chapter 4), may be used for insomnia. For short-term use, benzodiazepines have the advantage of being relatively safe and effective. Long-term use can be habit-forming.

These medicines differ in how long they remain in the body (Figure 15). Short-acting medicines have the advantage of causing less daytime hangover or confusion. Long-acting sleeping pills may help relieve daytime anxiety.

Barbiturates

These medicines are discussed in Chapter 4. They are extremely addicting and are no longer recommended for the treatment of insomnia.

Chloral Hydrate

This medicine is very safe and effective. Unfortunately, tolerance develops so that it can be used for only a few days.

Figure 15.   **Benzodiazepine Sleeping Pills**

Shorter Acting

- Alprazolam (Xanax)
- Lorazepam (Ativan)
- Oxazepam (Serax)
- Temazepam (Restoril)
- Triazolam (Halcion)

Longer Acting

- Chlorazepate (Tranxene)
- Chlordiazepoxide (Librium)
- Diazepam (Valium)
- Flurazepam (Dalmane)
- Prazepam (Centrax)

Antihistamines

> Medicines in this section include the following:
>
> - Diphenhydramine (Benadryl)
> - Promethazine (Phenergan)
> - Hydroxyzine (Atarax, Vistaril)

Some of the antihistamines are available over-the-counter as sleeping pills; others require a prescription. These medicines are generally effective and safe. However, they may cause anticholinergic side effects (see Chapter 3) that can lead to serious complications in some older people.

QUESTION: What about chronic insomnia that doesn't go away after short-term treatment?

ANSWER: Depending on the cause, the treatment of chronic insomnia varies. In most cases, a prescription for sleeping pills is not a first step. First, your doctor may have you keep a chart or diary of your sleep problems. He or she may then recommend some changes in your sleeping habits or evening activities. Furthermore, your doctor may refer you to a *sleep laboratory* for overnight evaluation of your sleeping difficulty. Based on the findings of a sleep evaluation, your doctor will better be able to recommend an effective treatment for you. Often this involves ways to improve your sleep hygiene. For certain rare forms of sleep apnea, however, your doctor might recommend surgery to improve breathing during sleep.

Some psychiatrists prescribe sedating antidepressant medicines for chronic insomnia. Usually, lower doses than are needed to treat depression are sufficient to improve sleep.

Used this way, some antidepressants are safe and effective for longer use since no tolerance to these medicines develops. Another helpful strategy is the use of a nonprescription medicine called L-tryptophan. This naturally occurring chemical, found in high concentration in milk, is converted by the body to a biochemical in the brain known to bring about sleep. This chemical is partly responsible for the effectiveness of drinking warm milk before retiring.

QUESTION: What is "sundowning" and how is it treated?

ANSWER: Sundowning (see Figure 14) is not true insomnia. It is a disturbance of sleep caused by severe evening agitation. Treatment of this condition with sleeping pills—a mistake commonly made by physicians not trained as psychiatrists or as geriatricians—often only makes things worse. Sundowning is frequently improved where feasible by the discontinuation or reduction in dose of other medicines that may cause confusion as a side effect. Improving orientation by leaving on the light and the television or radio in the evening may help. When medication is required, neuroleptic medicines are the most effective. Under these circumstances, they may be prescribed in very low doses to be taken around dinner time (see Chapter 6 for further details).

Although difficulty in falling asleep is a very common complaint of older people, it is a complicated problem that, when severe, requires careful medical attention. Sleeping pills may be helpful for short periods of use during severe stress or physical illness. However, if your insomnia persists and you are still taking sleeping pills, you *may* have a bigger problem than you started out with. Again, *the indiscriminate use of sleeping pills is medically unsafe.* If you feel you need further help, see your psychiatrist or other physician trained in the diagnosis and treatment of sleep problems.

CHAPTER 6

The Use of Medications in Treating Severe Agitation, Disturbed Thinking, and Disturbed Behavior

In this chapter we discuss medicines used to treat disturbances of thinking and behavior (Figure 16). Although other forms of therapy are important in the treatment of these disorders, our intent here is to discuss treatment with medicine. If you have decided to read only this chapter, then we recommend that you review Chapters 1 and 2 as well.

Symptoms of severe agitation, irrational thinking, and disturbed be-

Figure 16.   **Medicines Used to Treat Severe Agitation, Disturbed Thinking, and Disturbed Behavior**

- Chlorpromazine (Thorazine)
- Fluphenazine (Prolixin)
- Haloperidol (Haldol)
- Loxapine (Loxitane)
- Mesoridazine (Serentil)
- Molindone (Moban)
- Perphenazine (Trilafon)
- Pimozide (Orap)
- Thioridazine (Mellaril)
- Thiothixene (Navane)
- Trifluoperazine (Stelazine)

havior have numerous causes. Such symptoms often appear in psychiatric disorders such as **schizophrenia**, **mania**, severe **depression**, **Alzheimer's disease** (and related disorders), and **delirium**. Many physical illnesses that affect older people can produce these symptoms as well. These illnesses can include stroke, brain tumors, seizure disorders (epilepsy), thyroid disease, diabetes, heart disease, infections, and others. Intoxication with or withdrawal from prescription and nonprescription drugs or alcohol can also cause such symptoms. They also may be experienced during recovery from surgery or periods of treatment in intensive care units. Therefore, when an older person develops these symptoms, a thorough medical evaluation—including physical examination and appropriate laboratory tests—is needed to learn the cause(s) and to guide treatment.

Psychiatrists often prescribe **neuroleptic medicines** for the treatment of disturbed thinking and behavior. Especially when these symptoms are associated with frightening distortions of reality or bizarre or violent behavior, neuroleptics may be useful. When these symptoms are the predominant emotional problem, the neuroleptic

medicines often are effective in relieving symptoms, regardless of the cause.
Neuroleptics reduce agitation, hostility, and combative behavior and often
relieve **hallucinations** and delusions. A
hallucination is a false experience,
such as hearing voices talk to you
when nobody is there or seeing visions
of things that are not there. Psychiatrists use the word *psychosis* to refer to
many conditions in which people experience such symptoms. When psy-
chotic symptoms are caused by physical diseases, physicians will prescribe
the specific treatment for the physical
ailment in addition to neuroleptics.

Initiation of treatment with neuroleptic medicines may lead to rapid
relief of agitation, combativeness, and
other disturbed behaviors within hours
or days. Other symptoms, such as delusions, hallucinations, and irrational
thinking, may take longer to improve
(days or weeks). Higher doses may be
associated with more side effects that

may be especially troublesome for older patients. Your doctor generally will find the lowest dose of the medicine that provides effective relief. Many very effective neuroleptic medicines currently are available for use, though they differ both in potency or strength (how many milligrams you have to take for the same effect) and in the side effects they can cause. Low-milligram-dosage medicines may have different side effects from high-milligram-dosage medicines. Your doctor will select a medicine and dose for your individual circumstances. Figure 17 lists neuroleptic medicines according to dosage.

QUESTION: What are the side effects of neuroleptic medicines?

ANSWER: The neuroleptics commonly produce different types of side effects. A group of side effects that af-

Figure 17. **Neuroleptic Medicines**

Low Milligrams	Middle Milligrams	High Milligrams
• Fluphenazine (Prolixin)	• Loxapine (Loxitane)	• Chlorpromazine (Thorazine)
• Haloperidol (Haldol)	• Mesoridazine (Serentil)	• Thioridazine (Mellaril)
• Perphenazine (Trilafon)	• Molindone (Moban)	
• Pimozide (Orap)		
• Thiothixene (Navane)		
• Trifluoperazine (Stelazine)		

fect bodily movements is unique to this class of medicines. This group, medically referred to as **extra-pyramidal side effects**, deserves special attention.

Extrapyramidal Side Effects
(Movement-Related Side Effects)

Parkinsonism

This group is so named because of the similarity these side effects have to the symptoms experienced by patients with Parkinson's disease. However, *neuroleptic medications do not cause Parkinson's disease.* These symptoms include slowness of movement, decreased facial expression, stiffness, shaking, stooped posture, shuffling, and drooling. When parkinsonism is mild, it may be barely noticeable and easily tolerated. When more severe, however, these side effects require their own treatment. If possible, the psychiatrist might lower the dose of the neuroleptic medicine. Alternatively, it may be helpful to add an anti-parkinson medicine (e.g., benztropine mesylate [Cogentin]). These medicines are commonly used for the treatment of the early stages of Parkinson's disease and are very effective in reducing the parkinsonian side effects of neuroleptics. Unfortunately, most anti-parkinson medicines are capable of producing anticholinergic side effects that are particularly troublesome for older patients. (Anticholinergic side effects are discussed later in this chapter.) Sometimes, anticholinergic side effects limit the usefulness of antiparkinson medications in older patients. A unique antiparkinson drug, amantadine (Symmetrel), does not produce anticholinergic symptoms. Some psychiatrists feel that amantadine (Symmetrel) may be a good alternative for older patients. If all else fails, and you clearly need to take a neuroleptic drug, your doctor might try switching to a different medicine.

Akathisia

Neuroleptic medicines may produce an uncomfortable sense of restlessness, called akathisia by psychiatrists. With akathisia, there is a strong urge to move around, making it hard to remain still, and leading to tension or agitation. Such side effects can go unrecognized by physicians not specially trained in this area. Akathisia may be mistaken for a worsening of the original diagnosed agitation or disturbed behavior, and be treated incorrectly. The antiparkinson medicines may be helpful in relieving this problem. Other medicines such as the anti-anxiety drugs (Chapter 4) or propranolol (Inderal) are also sometimes helpful in relieving akathisia.

Dystonic Reaction

A dystonic reaction is a sudden, severe muscle cramp or spasm that may occur within the first hours or days of neuroleptic treatment, but rarely after that. Fortunately, it is less common than the other movement-related side effects and rare among older patients. The spasms may affect the neck, tongue, arms, or other parts of the body and can be very uncomfortable and frightening. Dystonic reactions do respond rapidly to treatment with antiparkinson medicine. The treatment—an injection of one of the antiparkinson medicines—usually relieves the muscle spasms within minutes. If you experience a sudden or severe dystonic reaction, you should call your doctor immediately or go directly to a hospital emergency room.

Tardive Dyskinesia

Tardive dyskinesia, unlike other movement-related side effects of neuroleptic medicines, usually does not occur until after years of neuroleptic treatment. Tardive dyskinesia is abnormal twitching or writhing movements that most commonly affect the face and tongue, although the arms, legs, torso, and other parts of the body may also be affected. Some patients find these abnormal movements not only embarrassing, but impairing.

Tardive dyskinesia is a more serious movement-related side effect of neuroleptic medicine both because it doesn't respond to treatment and because it may be long-lasting or permanent in some people. The only current effective treatment is to stop the use of neuroleptic medicine; thereafter, improvement may take several months or longer. However, for some patients, it may be necessary to continue taking the neuroleptic medicine to prevent behavioral symptoms from returning, posing a significant treatment problem for doctor and patient alike. Although tardive dyskinesia occurs only in about 20 percent of patients taking neuroleptics for prolonged periods, older people are more sensitive to medicine and therefore at greater risk to develop this problem.

QUESTION: These side effects sound terrible; why do doctors prescribe medicines that may cause permanent problems?

ANSWER: Despite the risks, neuroleptics are the safest and most effective group of medicines to treat extremely disturbed, irrational, or agitated behavior. Doctors prescribe medicines by balancing their benefits against their potential risks. Research is currently underway to discover neuroleptics that do not produce movement-related side effects, but as yet, none are available for routine use.

When doctors prescribe neuroleptic medicines, they ordinarily take certain precautions. First, the doctor will often prescribe the lowest effective dose. Second, during the course of treatment, the doctor will check you periodically to detect early signs of abnormal movements. Finally, after prolonged neuroleptic treatment, the doctor probably will discuss with you the possibility of lowering the dosage or halting the medicine to see if it is still needed. With these precautions, neuroleptic medicines provide safe and effective relief of symptoms for many patients with severe disorders.

Neuroleptic medicines produce other side effects unrelated to bodily movement. Anticholinergic side effects, mentioned before, are an important group of side effects common to other classes of medicines, such as some antidepressants and antiparkinson medicines. Anticholinergic side effects are caused by the medicine's effect on a natural and normal chemical—acetyl choline—found throughout the body. Because this chemical is important for the function of most of the organs of the body, the symptoms produced by medicines with anticholinergic side effects are diverse. Anticholinergic side effects usually are only a nuisance. However, older patients may be more sensitive to such side effects, that, if severe, may require medical intervention. The anticholinergic side effects are listed in Figure 18.

Other Side Effects

Neuroleptic medicine may affect the blood pressure reflexes, causing low blood pressure leading to light-headedness, unsteadiness, or dizziness when standing. Because this may increase an older patient's risk of falling, careful blood pressure monitoring is required. If light-headedness is a problem, you can take certain helpful steps. First, be sure to arise very slowly from a lying or sitting position; be sure you have your equilibrium before walking away from sources of support. Second, ask your doctor whether support stockings might be of help to you. If you are already taking medicine for treatment of high blood pressure and treatment with a neuroleptic causes you to be light-headed, your doctor may be able to correct the problem by lowering or stopping your blood pressure medicine.

Neuroleptics may cause drowsiness. In this case, your doctor may have you take the medicine in one dose before bed. Other possible side effects include sweating and sensitivity to sunburn. As a precaution against

Figure 18. **Anticholinergic Side Effects**

Common side effects that, if persistent, should be reported to your doctor:

- Dry mouth—can lead to dental problems or loose-fitting dentures
- Blurred vision—may interfere with reading
- Constipation—responds to high fiber diet, fluids, exercise
- Rapid heartbeat—should be monitored in people with heart disease
- Mild difficulty urinating—may be a particular problem for people with enlarged prostate gland

Rare side effects that should be reported to your doctor immediately:

- Eye pain—medicine with anticholinergic effects may aggravate narrow angle type glaucoma
- Irregular heartbeat
- Skin rash
- Extreme difficulty starting urine or total inability to urinate
- Abdominal pain or distention
- Confusion, hallucinations, agitation, forgetfulness

severe sunburn, sunscreens with the ingredient PABA or other sun-blocking substances should be used by people using neuroleptic medication.

QUESTION: All these side effects make neuroleptic treatment seem complicated. Are some neuroleptics better than others for the elderly?

ANSWER: Many geriatric psychiatrists recommend beginning with a low milligram type of neuroleptic medication (see Figure 17). These medicines cause the lowest anticholinergic side effects, produce somewhat less drowsiness, and have the least effect on blood pressure and the heart. Unfortunately, they are the highest in movement-related side effects. The high milligram (low potency) neuroleptics produce little effect on bodily movements, but are much more likely to cause troublesome anticholinergic symptoms or light-

headedness. Sometimes, a little trial
and error is necessary to find the particular medicine which is best for a
particular individual. Neuroleptic
medicines are generally quite safe
when prescribed by physicians knowl-
edgeable in their use.

QUESTION: What if the original
symptoms of disturbed behavior and
irrational thinking don't improve after
a few weeks?

ANSWER: If you don't seem to improve, your doctor may try raising the
dose of your medication or may
switch to a different medicine. Once
you do improve, it may be possible
for your doctor to lower the dose
somewhat and to simplify your dose
schedule. Since these medicines often
can be taken once a day, it may be
easier and more effective to take the
entire dose either just after you wake

or immediately before bed in the evening.

QUESTION: For how long do you have to keep taking neuroleptic medicine once you improve?

ANSWER: That depends on the problem. For a temporary period of agitation or confusion during a physical illness, a short course of treatment may be sufficient. On the other hand, after an episode of schizophrenia, mania, or severe depression with delusions, prolonged maintenance therapy for months or years may be necessary to prevent relapse.

QUESTION: Why are some patients prescribed fluphenazine decanoate (Prolixin-D) shots?

ANSWER: Fluphenazine decanoate (Prolixin-D) is an example of a **depot medicine**. A depot medicine is given by injection and then small amounts are released slowly from the injection site into the body. It can be given as often as once a week or as infrequently as once every six weeks, although once every two to three weeks is a schedule often prescribed. Depot medicines substitute for oral medicine and are advantageous for people who are unable to take pills regularly. The injection helps to make sure that these people are receiving the medicine they need. Until recently, fluphenazine decanoate (Prolixin-D) was the only depot neuroleptic available. Not too long ago, a depot form of haloperidol (Haldol) also became available.

QUESTION: What happens if you abruptly stop taking neuroleptic medicine?

ANSWER: Neuroleptic medicines are not addicting or habit forming.

However, because the body can become used to the anticholinergic effects, some patients may experience *anticholinergic withdrawal symptoms*. These may include nausea and vomiting, cramps, diarrhea, nasal congestion, headache, chills, and goose flesh, lasting no longer than a few days. Anticholinergic withdrawal is not dangerous medically, but can be uncomfortable. Thus, as a precaution, it is better to go off neuroleptics gradually, under your doctor's supervision, than to stop taking them all at once.

Some Final Precautions

Neuroleptics add to the effects of alcohol, sleeping pills, and tranquilizers. Using combinations of these should be avoided, unless you are using them under a psychiatrist's careful supervision. If neuroleptics cause you to feel drowsy or less alert, you should avoid driving or using machinery. Finally, if you accidentally take an overdose of a neuroleptic medicine or think you may have taken one, seek medical attention immediately.

In conclusion, when used according to the directions of a doctor trained in the use of neuroleptics, these medicines help many people obtain relief from some of the most disturbing symptoms of severe psychiatric disorders.

CHAPTER 7

The Use of Medications in Treating Alzheimer's Disease and Related Forms of Dementia

In this chapter we discuss the emotional and behavioral symptoms associated with Alzheimer's disease and related disorders. Although our purpose is to focus on treatment with medicine, other forms of therapy are important. If you have decided to read only this chapter, we recommend that you review Chapters 1 and 2. In addition, reading other chapters on treatment of other problems might help you understand how psychiatric medicines are used to treat certain symptoms.

When asked the question, "What does 'senility' mean?" many people answer "'senility' means old age." The thought of senility makes many people, old and young, worried about their future. The word "senility" provokes anxiety because it has come to stand for two false beliefs about aging common in our culture. One is that senility is an inevitable part of aging. The other is that any mental or emotional disturbance in later life is due to senility. In this book, we have attempted to dispel these myths. We have also tried to point out that old people suffer from many of the same mental and emotional problems as younger people and respond just as well *if they receive the right treatment.*

In this chapter, we do not discuss a particular group of medicines. Rather, we attempt to clarify a few things about "senility" and explain what doctors can and cannot do to help. In this context, we talk about the role of treatment with medicine.

When we use the word "senility," we are referring to various forms of **dementia**. Dementia refers to any illness that leads to a deterioration of intellectual functions such as memory, language, and thinking. If progressive, it later leads to a loss of knowledge learned and, eventually, to difficulty in recognizing familiar people or things. Dementia can affect younger people, but it more commonly occurs in later life, when it is referred to as *senile dementia*. In this context, the word *senile* is defined as "occurring later in life" and comes from historical English language usage.

Dementia has many causes. In older patients, **Alzheimer's disease** is the most common case of dementia. Another major cause of dementia is the accumulated effect of multiple strokes. There are many other causes of dementia, including those caused by treatable physical diseases. In such cases, which are relatively rare, treatment may either improve the dementia or prevent it from growing worse. Therefore, it is extremely important for anyone who develops symptoms of dementia to have a thorough evaluation to make sure that a treatable form of dementia is not overlooked. Unfortunately, for the vast majority of patients with dementia today, there is no effective treatment for the intellectual decline. There is treatment, however, for the disturbances of mood and behavior that may accompany the intellectual decline.

QUESTION: Are there experimental treatments that show any promise?

ANSWER: Much research is being conducted at various research centers, but as yet, no treatment for intellectual decline has proven to be effective. The list of treatments that have been tried or are now under investigation

includes hydergine, physostigmine,
THA (tetrahydroaminoacridine), leci-
thin, GHA, acetyl choline, arecholine,
stimulants, hyperbaric oxygen,
gerovital, ACTH, and L-dopa. Some
of these are available; some physicians
prescribe them in the hope of obtain-
ing a limited benefit. Sometimes, it
simply helps for those involved to feel
that something is being done, but generally these treatments are not useful.
Occasionally, they can be harmful.

The medical profession has a long
tradition of caring for many patients
with illnesses for which there is no
currently known cure. The medical
specialty of psychiatry is uniquely
skilled to deal with many of the effects
of **Alzheimer's disease** and related
forms of dementia on both patients
and families. First, psychiatrists are
best qualified to recognize and diagnose other mental or emotional disorders in older people (Chapters 3–6)

that may be mistaken for dementia by other specialists. Moreover, because psychiatrists are physicians, they are able to identify physical problems, including medication side effects that may be contributing to an intellectual disturbance. Since psychiatrists are also trained in the various forms of psychotherapy and behavioral therapy, they may be able to assist patients and families to cope better with dementia, through the "talking treatment." Finally, even though there are no medicines that help the memory problem, psychiatrists may use some of the various **psychoactive medicines** to help relieve the emotional and behavioral disturbances that may occur in patients with dementia.

Dementia affects the function of many parts of the brain including the areas involved in emotions and control over behavior. Thus, in addition to the gradual intellectual decline, patients with dementia may experience disturbances of mood and behavior. Symptoms such as depression, confusion, hostility, agitation, combativeness, delusions, **hallucinations,** wandering, and sleep disturbances may appear. These symptoms are often relieved by treatment with the medicines used to treat such symptoms in patients without dementia (see Chapters 3–6). These emotional and behavioral symptoms can affect the quality of life for people with dementia as much as does the intellectual decline associated with these disorders. Therefore, dementia patients with such symptoms should receive psychiatric treatment when it is available. Research to develop better strategies to treat these distressing symptoms of dementia currently is being conducted by researchers in the subspecialty field of geriatric psychiatry and others.

GLOSSARY

Adverse medicine interactions: A result produced when two or more medicines (including over-the-counter medications) combine to produce a harmful effect.

Adverse reactions: Unexpected, sometimes harmful effects of a medicine. They are uncommon and generally not severe, but are unpredictable since they reflect the sensitivities of individuals instead of the typical action of the medicine.

Affective disorders: See **mood disorder** (Chapter 3).

Akathisia: A movement-related side effect of some medicines used in the treatment of severely disturbed behavior and thinking. This is experienced as an inner tension or physical restlessness which often causes a strong urge to pace (Chapter 6).

Alzheimer's disease: A disease of the brain resulting in disturbances of behavior, intellectual ability, and function that is a cause of many cases of senile dementia (Chapter 7).

Antianxiety medicines (see minor tranquilizers):   Medicines that relieve anxiety, an inner emotional state of nervousness, apprehension, or tension (Chapter 4).

Anticholinergic side effects: See Chapter 6.

Antidepressant medicines: Medicines often prescribed for the treatment of depressive illness (Chapter 3).

Antihistamines: Medicines commonly used to relieve itching and allergic symptoms. They may be used as well to relieve anxiety and are the active ingredients of some over-the-counter sleeping pills (Chapters 4 and 5).

Anxiety disorders: See Chapter 4.

Barbiturates: See Chapter 4.

Benzodiazepines: A family of medicines that is commonly used for sleeping and the relief of anxiety (Chapter 4). They are sometimes used in the treatment of movement-related side effects (Chapter 6).

Bipolar disorder (manic-depressive illness): See **mood disorder.**

Brand names: These are the particular names that pharmaceutical manufacturers give to the medicines they manufacture. Just like other products (corn flakes, facial tissues, gelatin, etc.), many medicines are made by more than one company, and thus each has a different brand name.

Delirium: A state of difficulty in thinking clearly that may be associated with disturbed thoughts and behavior. Although delirium resembles many psychiatric illnesses, it always is caused by a physical problem that must be identified and treated (Chapter 6).

Dementia: A condition in which people experience a loss of intellectual faculties and ability to take care of themselves. This is caused by diseases of the brain, most commonly **Alzheimer's disease** (Chapter 7).

Depot medicine: A medicine given by injection which slowly releases through the body over a period of time. It may be used in certain instances when patients are unable to remember to take medications for severe agitation (Chapter 6).

Depressive illness: A medical illness characterized by an abnormally severe and long lasting depressed mood that is out of proportion to circumstances in life (Chapter 3).

Detoxification: A medical treatment of weaning someone from a medicine or illegal drug upon which they are dependent.

Dose: The amount of medicine prescribed to be taken at one time.

Drug half-life: A property of medicines related to how long it takes them to clear out of the body.

Drug dependence: A state of emotional or physical addiction to a medicine which leads to a strong, sometimes unrealistic desire to keep taking the medicine.

Drug interaction: The effect one medicine may have on the action of another medication when both are being used at the same time.

Dystonic reaction: A muscle spasm sometimes caused by neuroleptic medicines (Chapter 6).

Electrocardiogram (EKG): A medical test in which the heart's natural electrical rhythm is recorded on paper through wires placed on the chest and limbs.

Electroconvulsive therapy (ECT): See Chapter 3.

Electroencephalogram (EEG): A medical test in which the brain's natural electrical waves (brain waves) are recorded on paper through wires placed on the scalp.

Extrapyramidal side effects: Movement-related side effects of neuroleptic medicines (Chapter 6).

Generic name: The chemical compound name for a medicine which is the same regardless of which pharmaceutical company manufactures the medicine (for example, gelatin is the generic name for Jello®).

Hallucination: A false sensory experience, such as hearing voices or seeing visions.

Hypertensive crisis: A dangerously high elevation of blood pressure that can result from failing to avoid certain foods or medicines while taking MAOI antidepressants (Chapter 3).

Hypnotic: A sleep-producing medicine often referred to as a sleeping pill (Chapter 5).

Insomnia: Difficulty or inability to sleep (Chapter 5).

Major tranquilizers: See **Neuroleptic medicines.**

Mania: A medical illness characterized by an extreme and prolonged abnormally happy or elated mood, as experienced by people with manic-depressive illness (Chapter 3).

Manic-depressive illness: See **Mood disorder.**

Milligram (mg): A measure of weight used to indicate the amount of a medicine. One ounce weighs about 3000 milligrams.

Minor tranquilizers (see also **Antianxiety medicines**): A group of medicines commonly prescribed for the relief of anxiety (Chapter 4).

Monoamine oxidase inhibitor: A particular class of antidepressant (Chapter 3).

Mood disorder: An illness that causes a prolonged disturbance of mood. This can take the form of abnormal depression or excessive happiness (Chapter 3).

Neuroleptic medicines: A group of medicines prescribed for the treatment of severe agitation or disturbed thinking or behavior (Chapter 6).

Neurotransmitters: Naturally occurring biochemicals in the brain that act as nerve signal messengers.

Organic brain syndrome: A disturbance of the brain affecting intelligence, emotions, or thinking, caused by a physical disease (Chapter 7).

Panic disorder: A medical illness in which people experience sudden severe spells of anxiety that come unexpectedly without a clear cause (Chapter 4).

Parkinsonism: A slowness of bodily movement associated with shaking, shuffling, and stiffness. This is one type of movement-related side effect of neuroleptic medicines (Chapter 6).

Psychoactive medication: Any medicine used to treat symptoms of mental or emotional problems. They include neuroleptics, antidepressants, lithium, antianxiety medicines, and sleeping pills.

Psychopharmacology: The science and clinical practice of using medication to relieve mental and emotional distress.

Psychosis: A state of mental illness in which thinking becomes irrational and disturbed (Chapter 6).

Psychotherapy (medical): A form of medical treatment for emotional disturbances in which better understanding and solutions to disorders are achieved through talking with a trained psychiatrist.

Schizophrenia: A type of medical illness with severe disturbance of thinking and behavior (Chapter 6).

Sedation: An action from a medicine that causes a calming, relaxing, or sleep-producing effect.

Sedative-hypnotic: A medication used predominantly for the treatment of anxiety or insomnia (Chapters 4 and 5).

Side effect: Undesirable, inconvenient, or occasionally harmful effects that all medicines may have at times.

Sundowning: The occurrence of severe agitation or confusion in the evening hours in otherwise relatively calm people (Chapter 5).

Tardive dyskinesia: A side effect of neuroleptic medications that causes abnormal twitching movements of the body (Chapter 6).

Therapeutic effect: The curative or helpful effect of a medication, such as relieving pain, lowering blood pressure, fighting infection, or relieving depression.

Tolerance: The tendency for some medicines to lose some of their effectiveness once the body gets accustomed to them.

Toxicity: The harmful effect of too much of a medicine.

Withdrawal symptoms: Physical and emotional symptoms experienced when people stop or are weaned off a medicine upon which they are dependent.

Index Of Medications